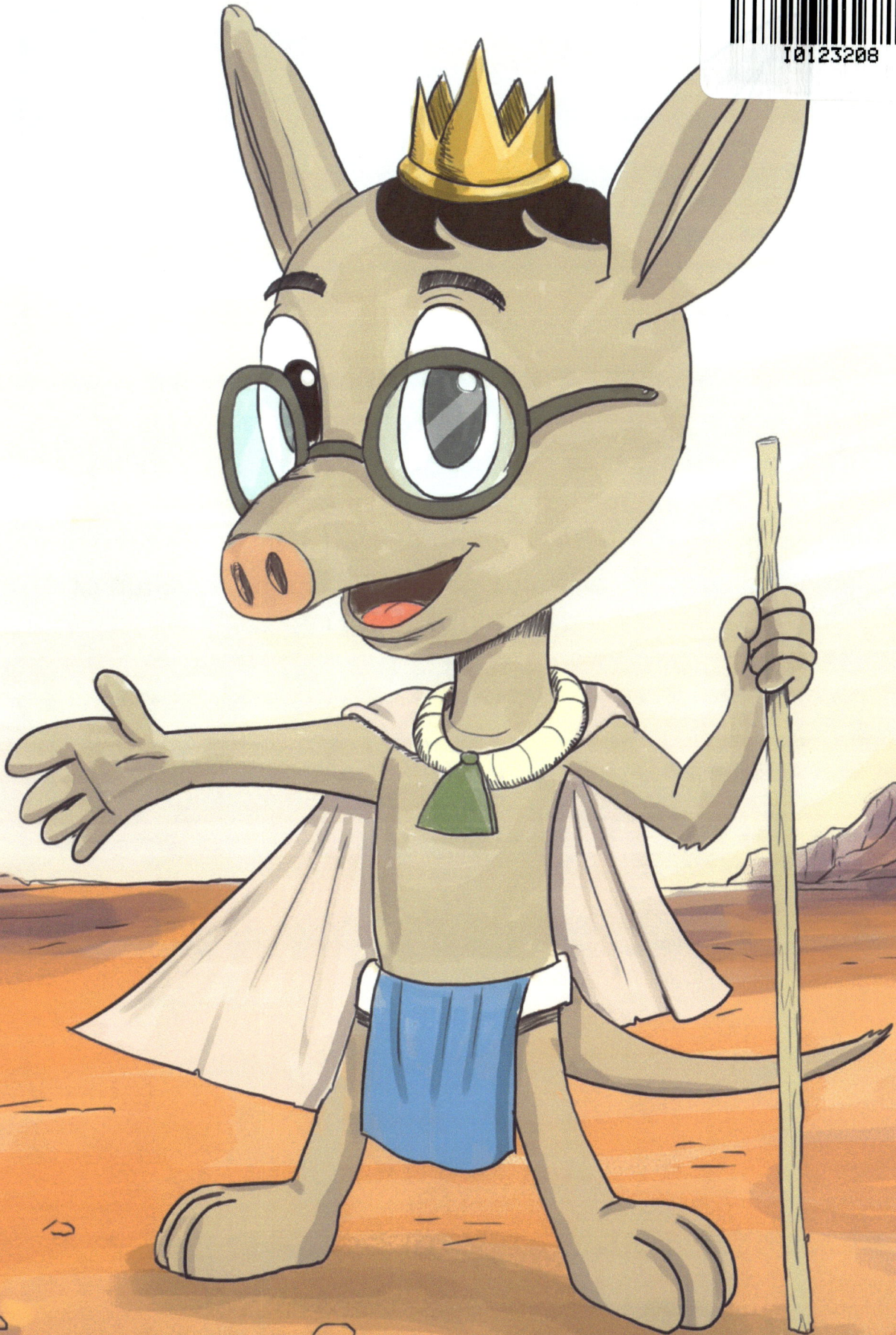

Ace The Aardvark
The King of Courage
Freezes His Fears of Textures

Writen by
Stacy Shaneyfelt

Illustrated by
Danko Herrera

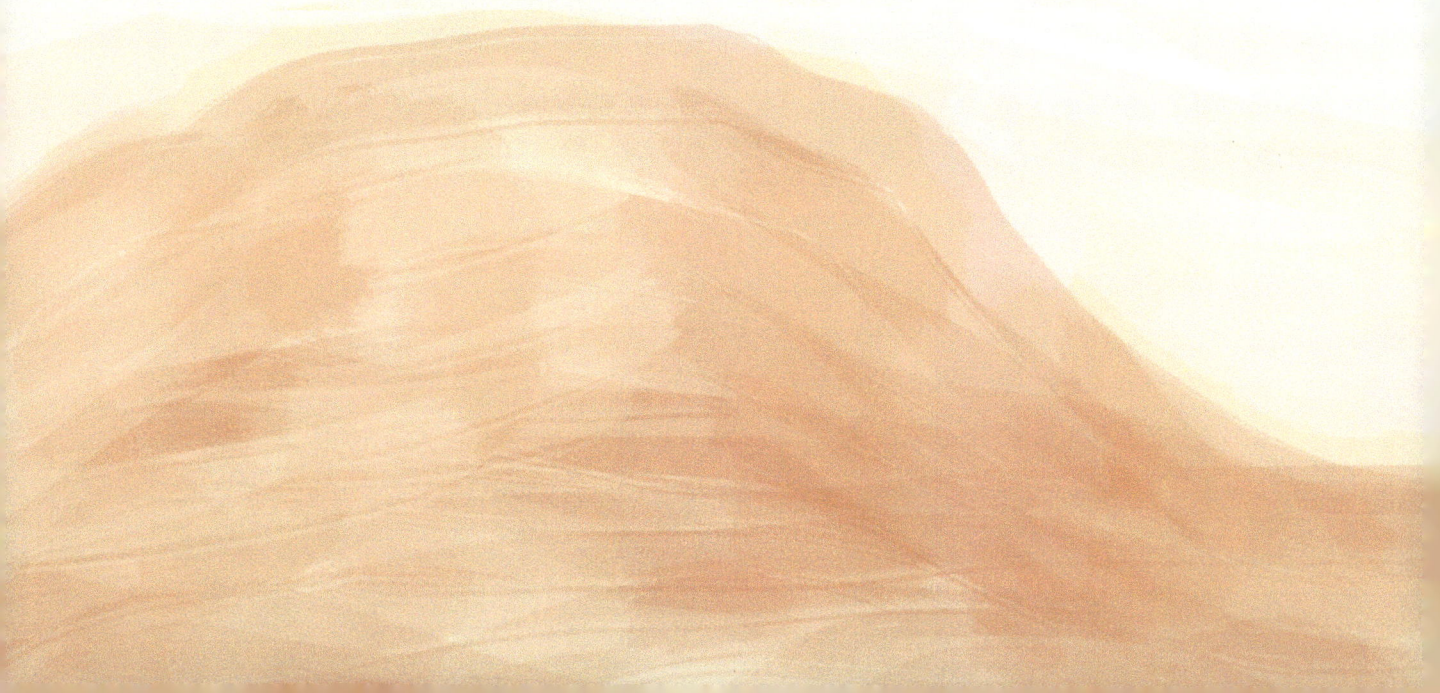

To my brave and beautiful daughters who "ace" their fears every day.

I love you with all my heart and shine my faith in you through the dark and lit moments of life!

I also extend a call to action to all sensory-processing

disorders, diagnoses, and challenges that so many

people endure.

May you find your "crown" of courage to cope and

calm.

To begin our tale, we visit Namibia's Damaraland. Ace the Aardvark snuggles joyfully in his burrow with his loving family.

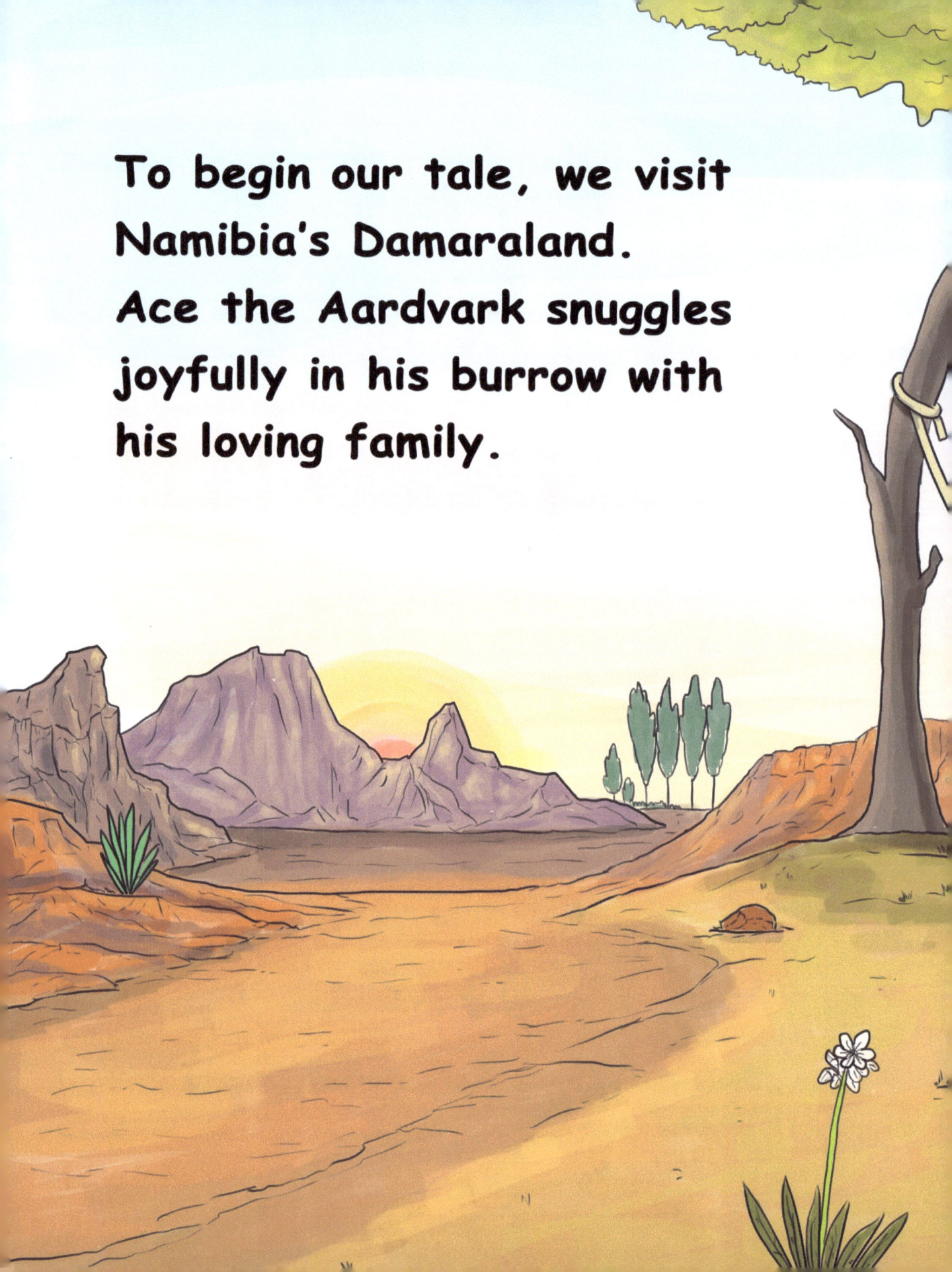

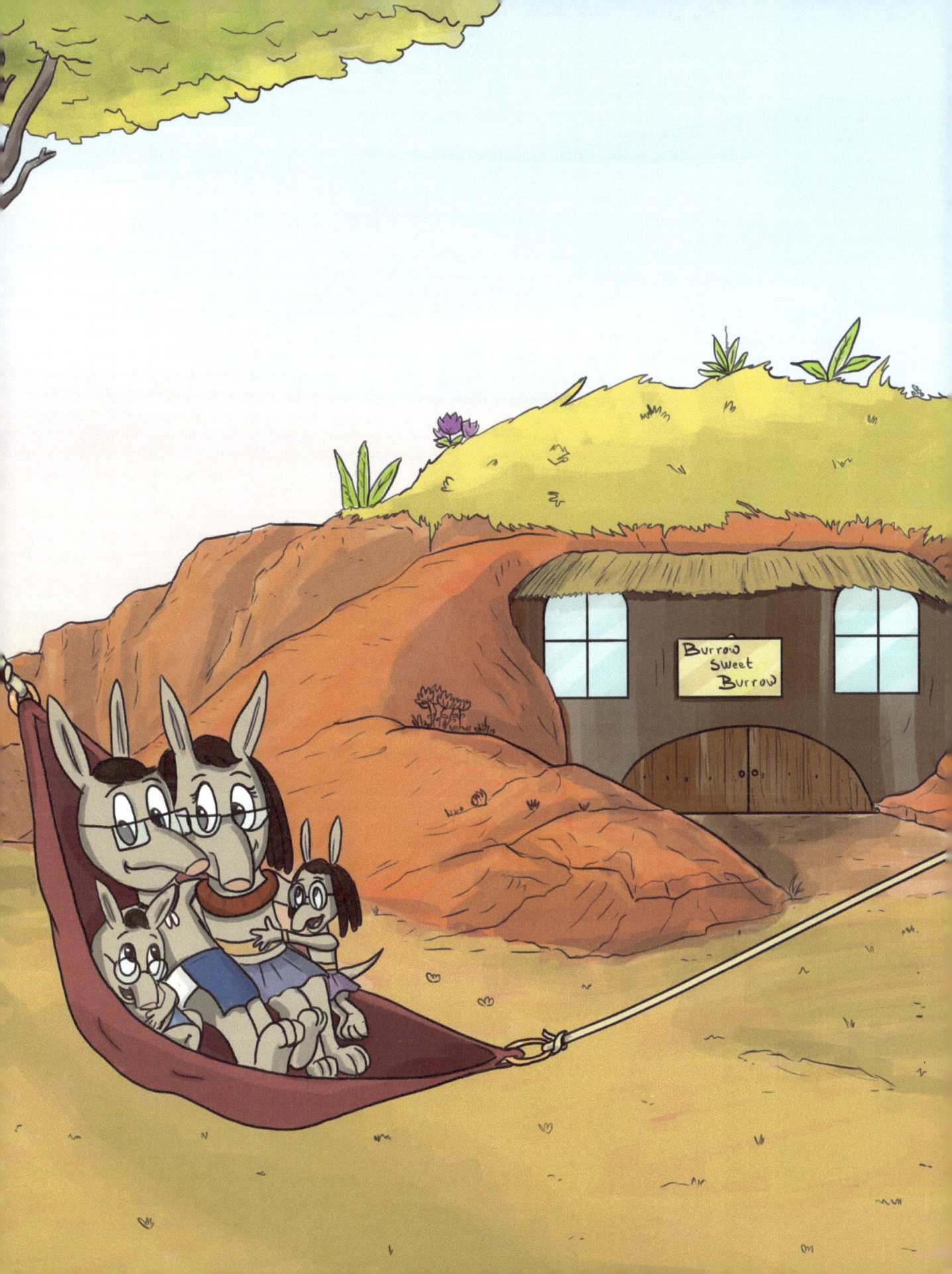

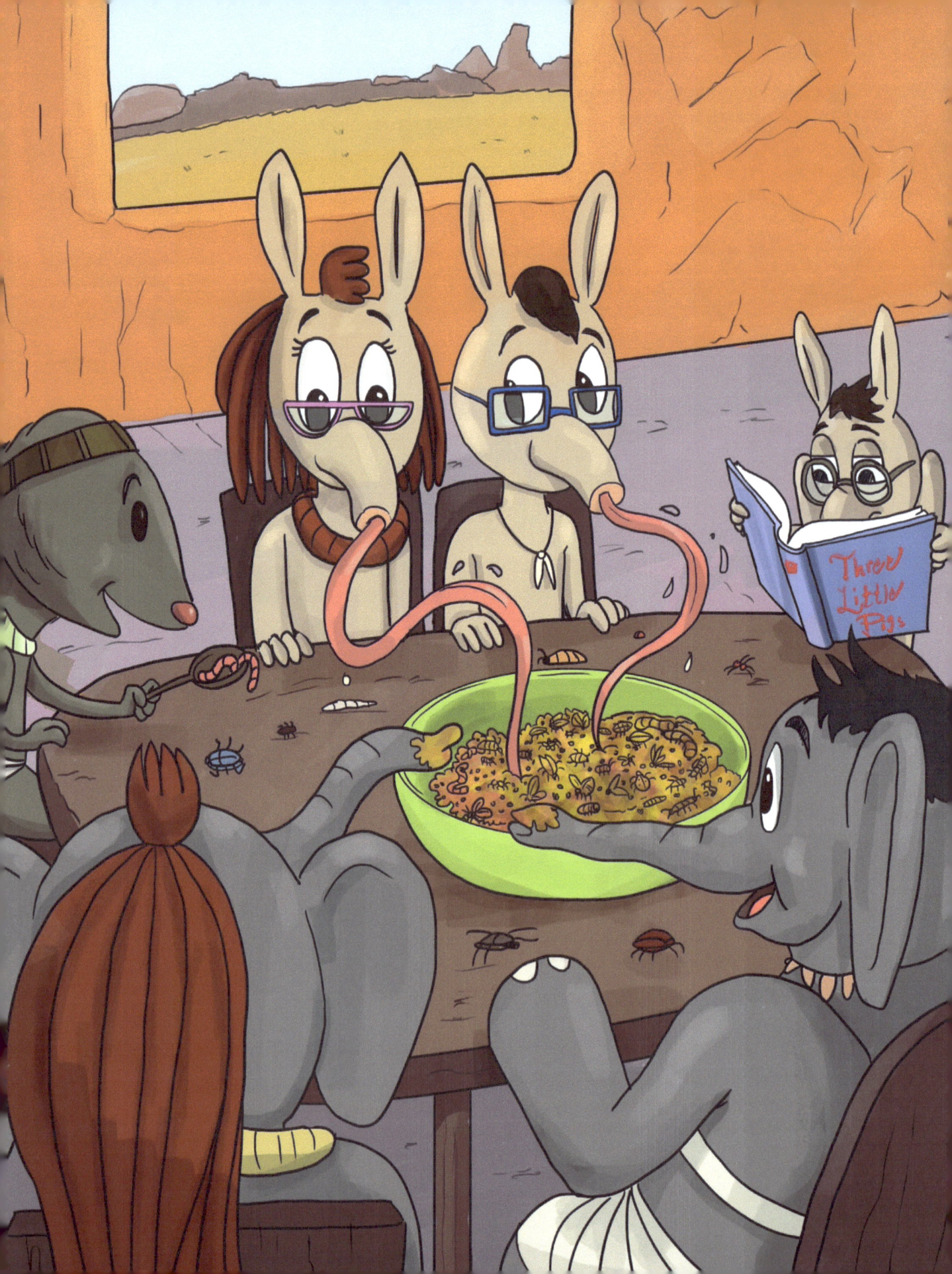

While he looks more like the fourth of the Three Little Pigs, this mini mammal is actually related to elephants and golden moles.

As the others gobble termite granola, Ace barely nibbles at the grainy bits, fearing its gritty texture like sawdust.

Right after breakfast, Ace first wants to play in the sand with Ayo and Ace's baby sister.

Yet when Ace grabs the shovel to dig, he fears the hot, scratchy sand scraping his ticklish toes!

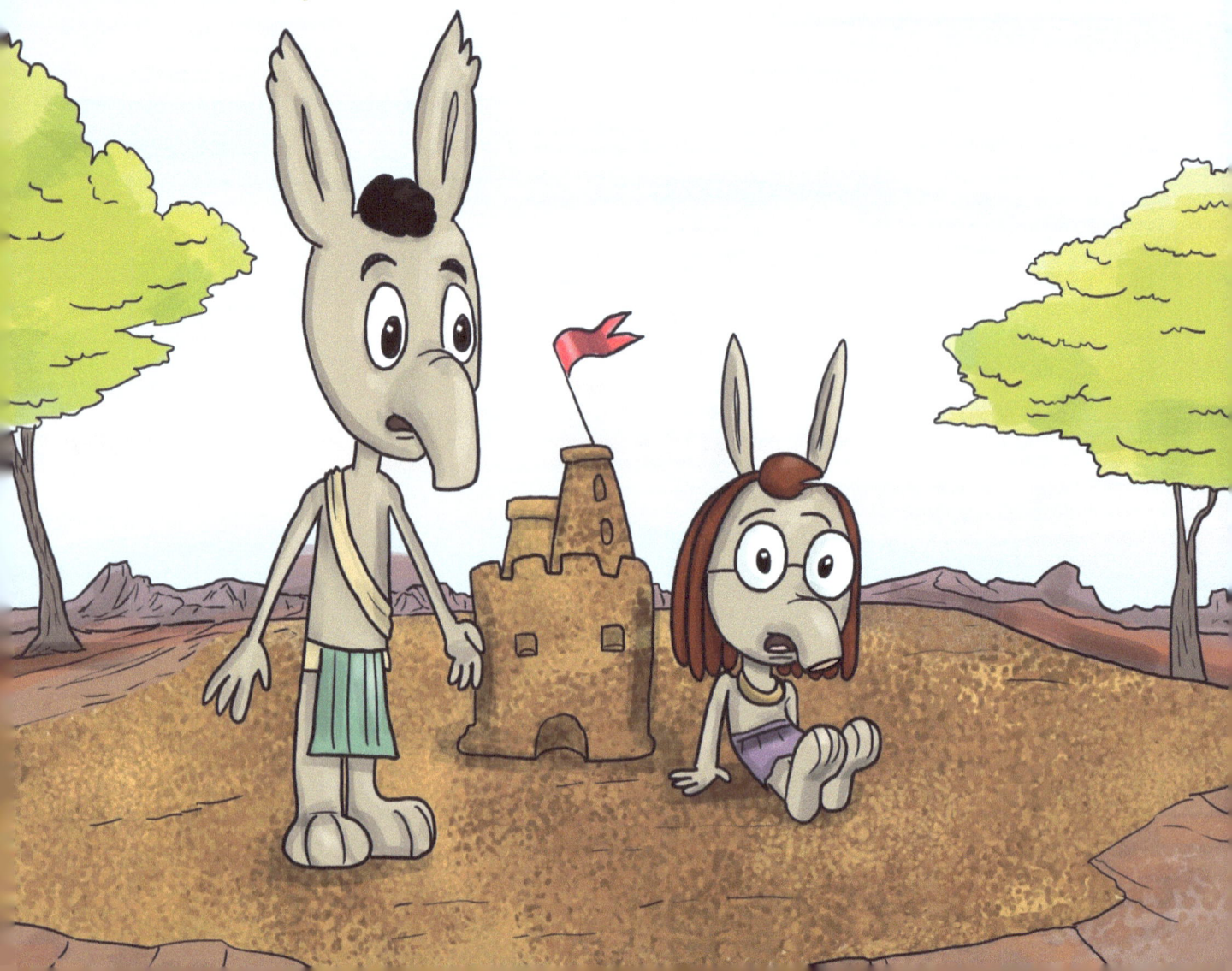

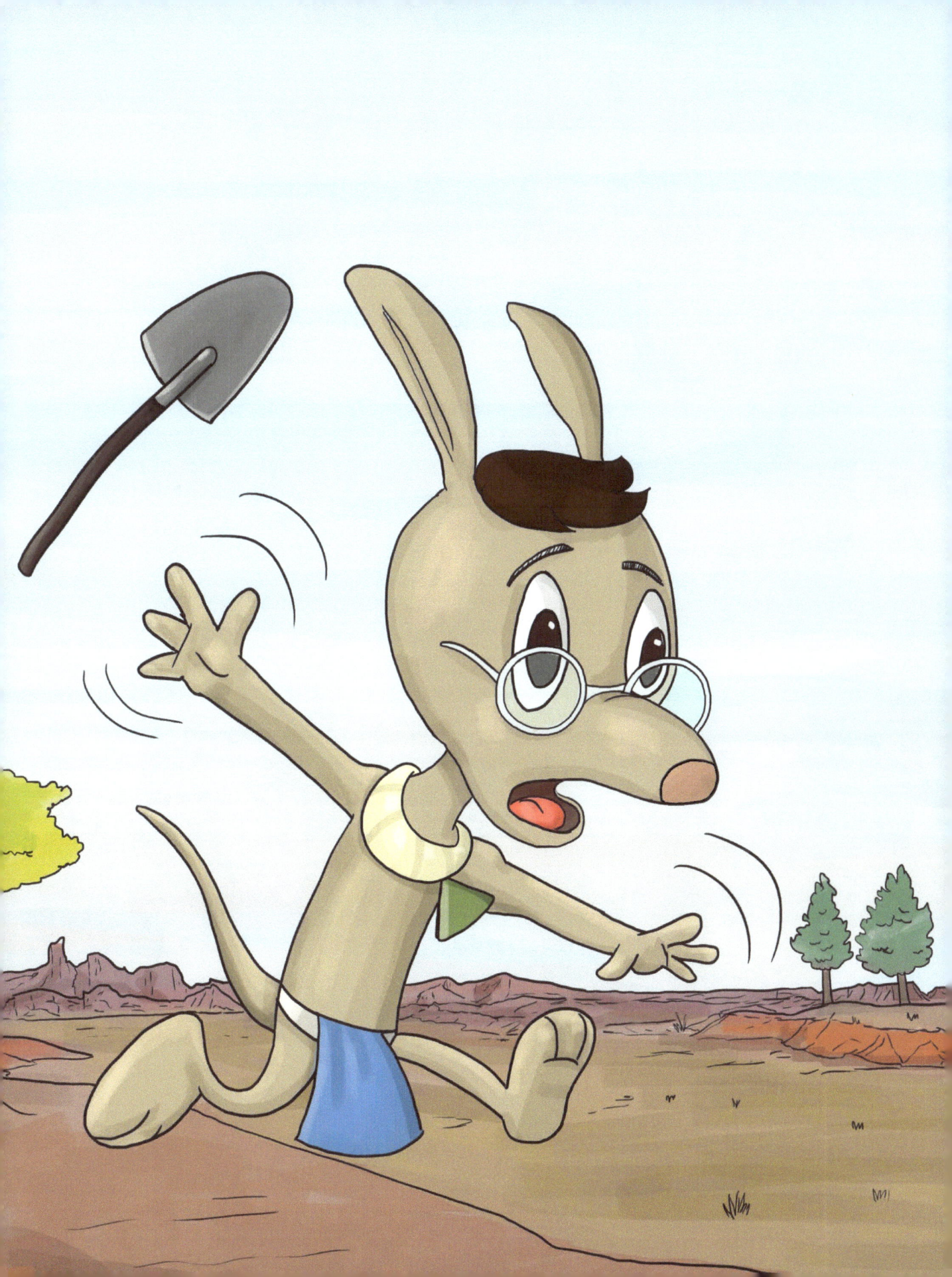

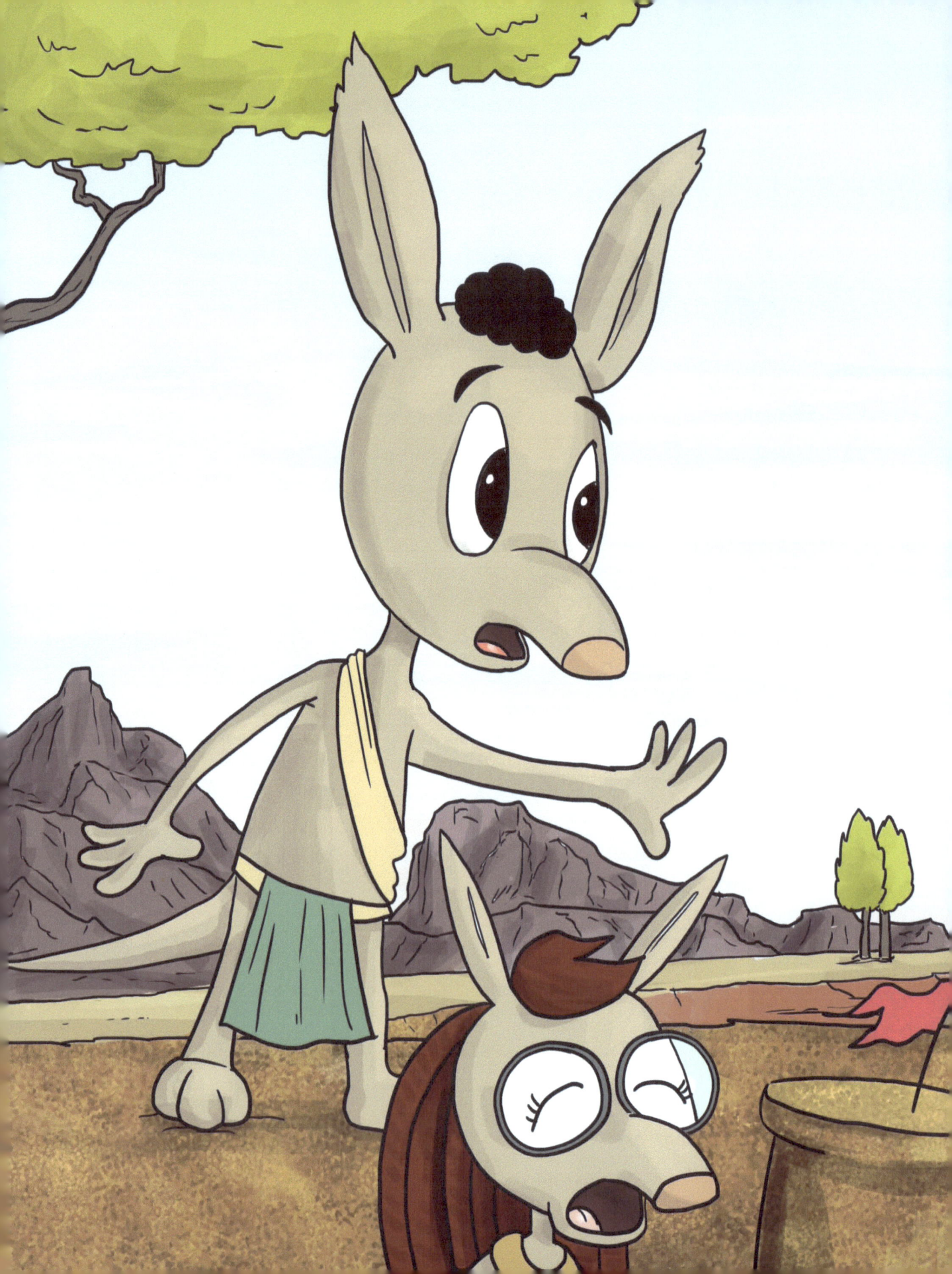

Instantly, Ayo begs, "Aw, come on, little buddy. The sun is bright today, so let's build our Royal Aardvark Kingdom!" Even baby Ava pleads with her brother.
But Ace's tummy grumbles as he screams,

It's the dungeon of dirt and sand that I don't like!
See you, Sir-Build-A Lot and Maiden Ava.
I'm heading back to my humble hammock!

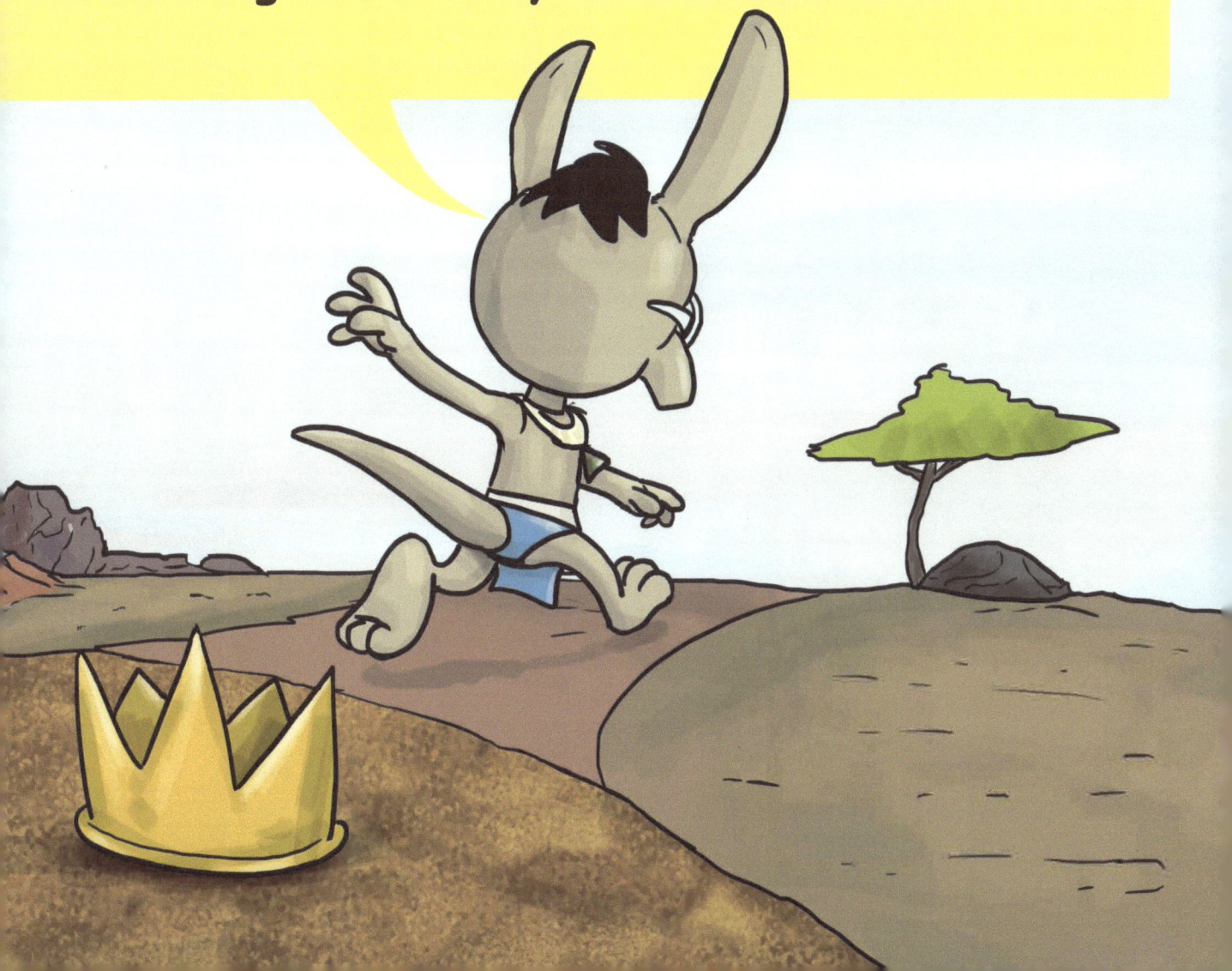

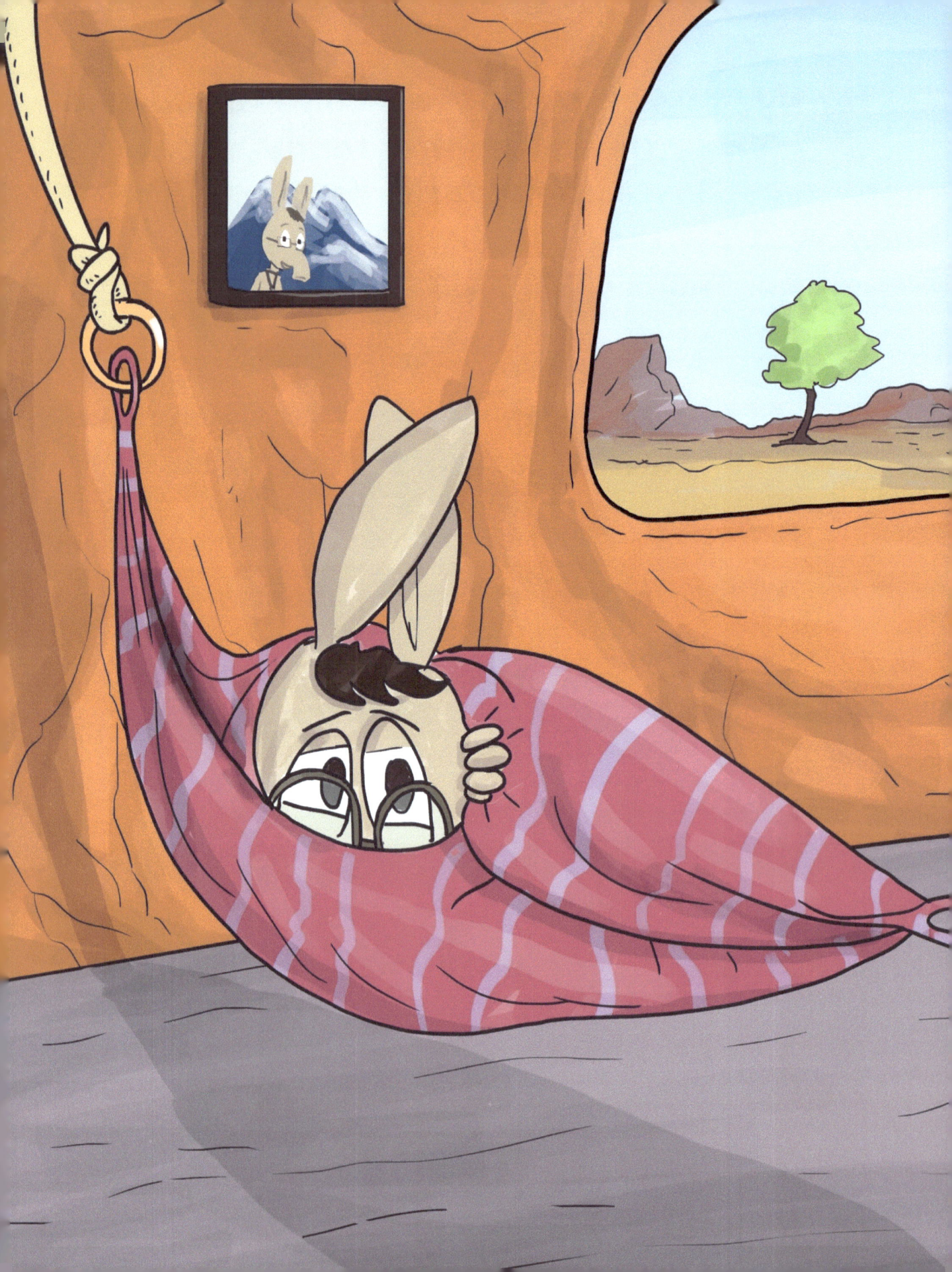

Following the sandcastle crash, Ace rocks back and forth, trying to freeze his fears and tears.

First, he does a negative thought stop that his teacher taught him.

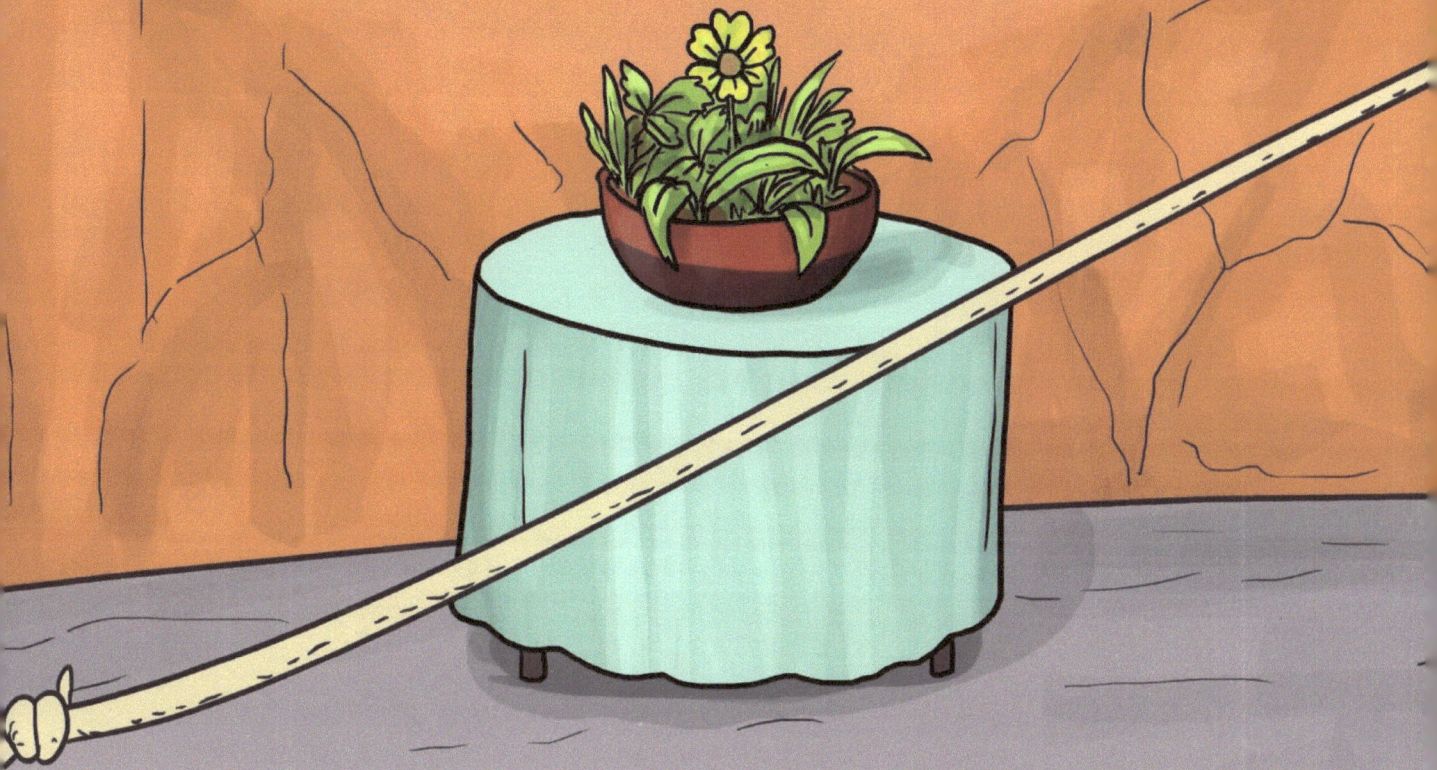

Like putting a lid on a bottle, he freezes his worries.

Meanwhile, Mama and Ava appear with soft smiles. Mama whispers,

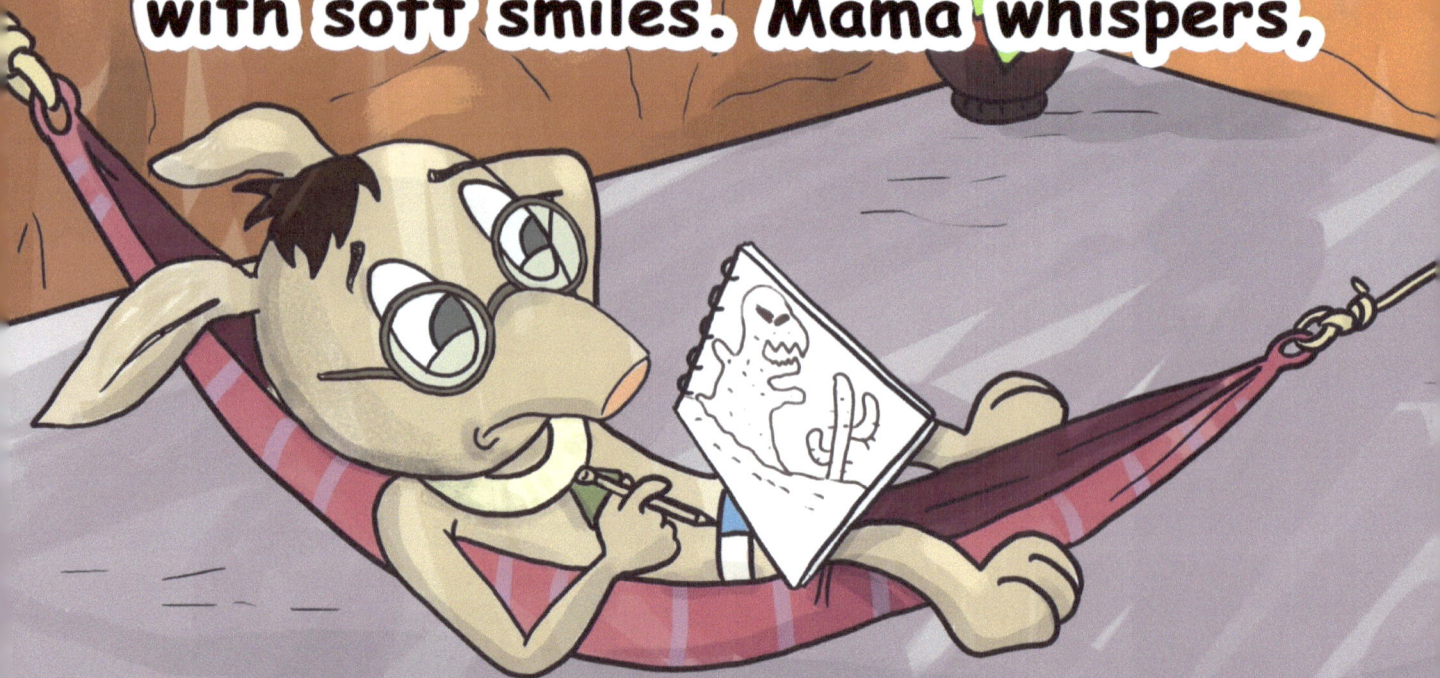

She draws her fear of aliens as Ace sketches his fear of sand and termite granola. Ava scribbles like a spider making a web.

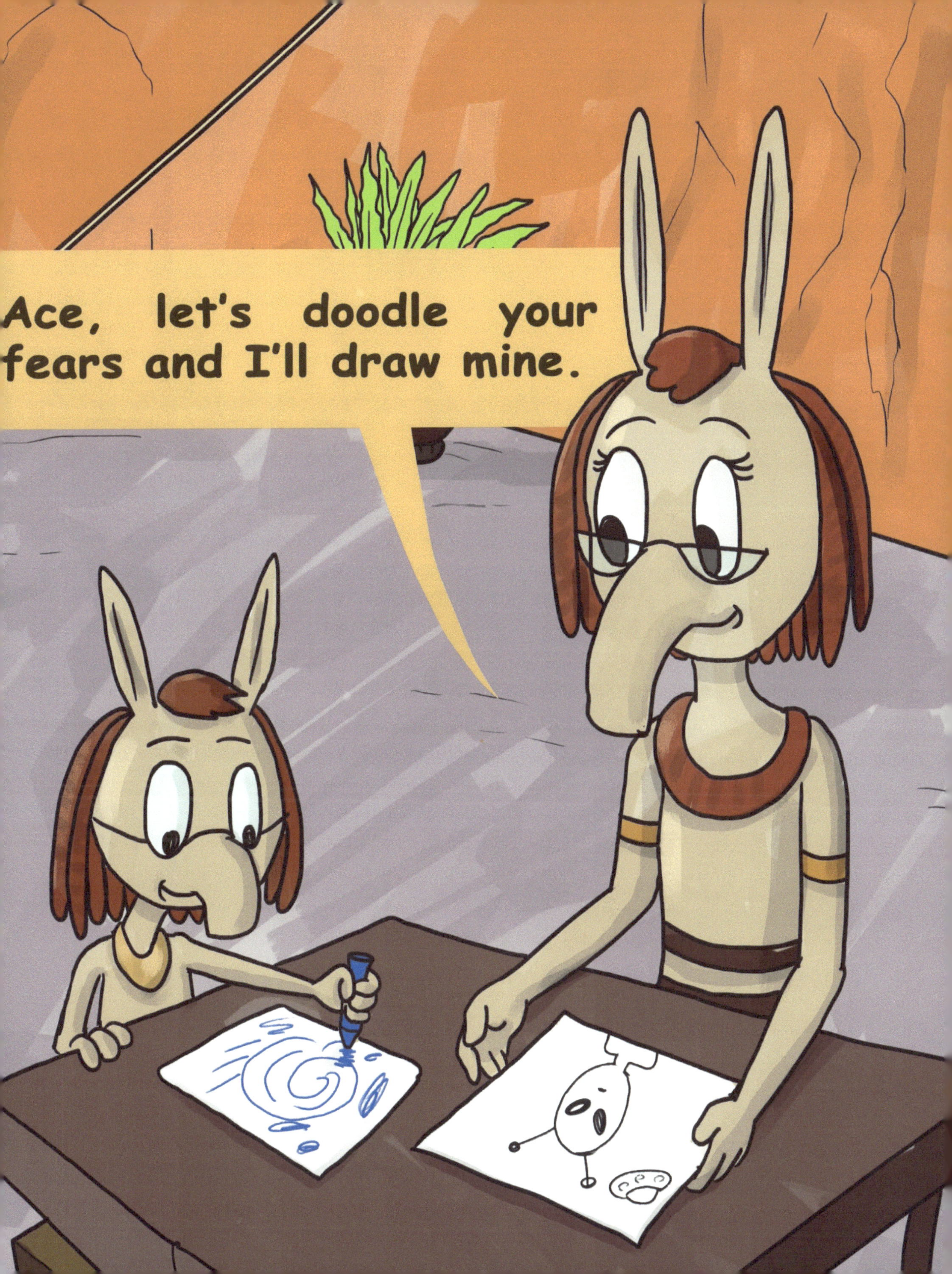
Ace, let's doodle your fears and I'll draw mine.

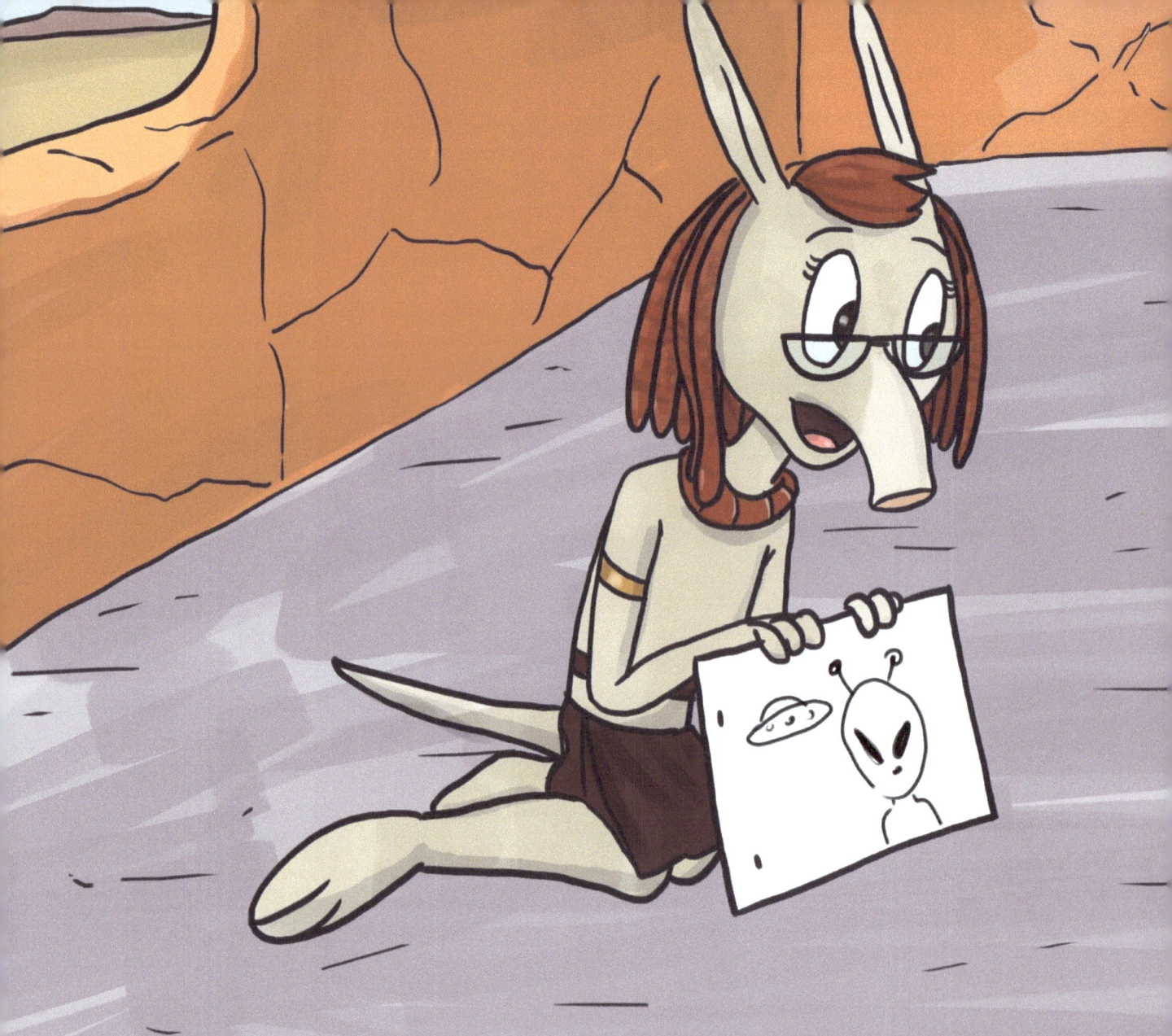

Next, Mama encourages Ace to talk about what he drew.
She models first, "I'm often scared that aliens will find our burrow, but I know our family protects our home. Plus, aliens only exist in meerkat movies, right?"

I drew my fear of sand and termite granola like a funny cactus robot!

Then it's Ace's turn to describe his art. He giggles, Ava chuckles and grins at her big brother's bravery to freeze his fears.

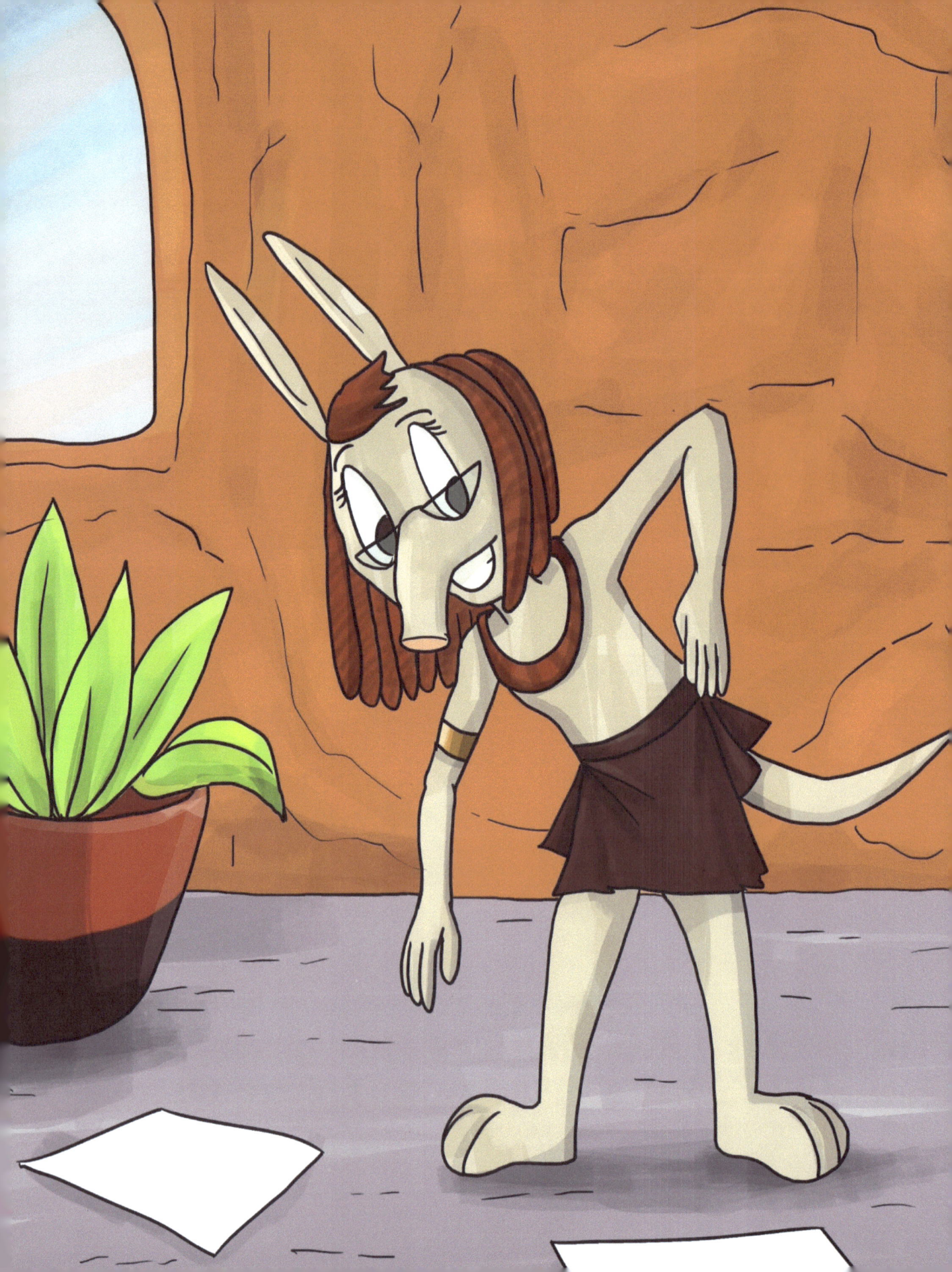

All at once, Ayo enters and they all break into a robot dance. Ayo shares his trick to conquer his fear of yetis. He adds,

I use the feelings versus facts game to check, is my fear based on a fact or a feeling?

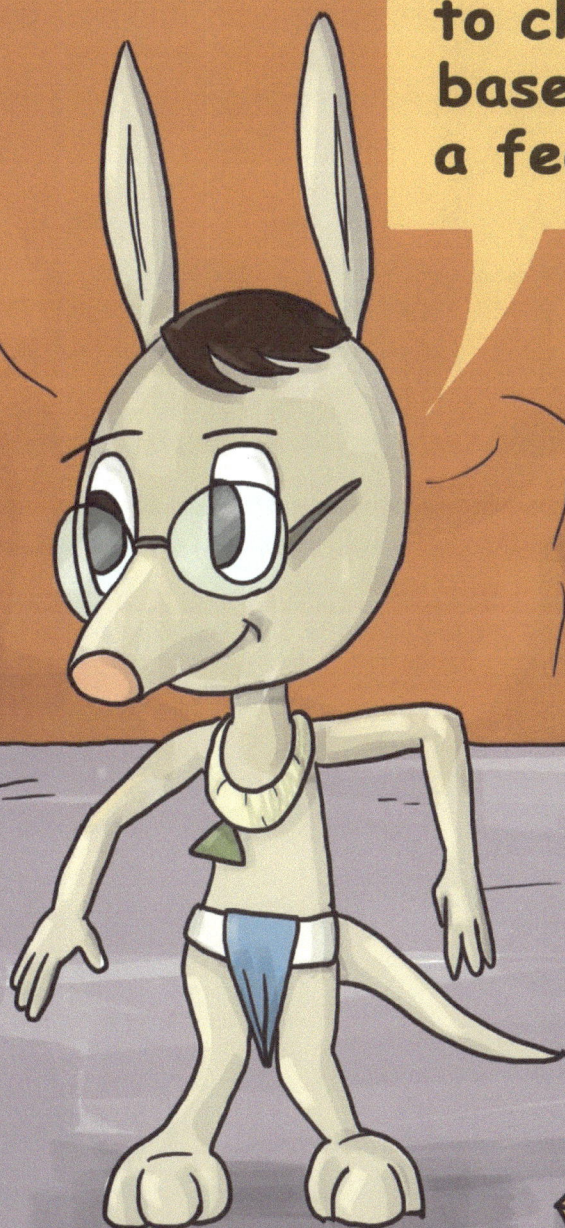

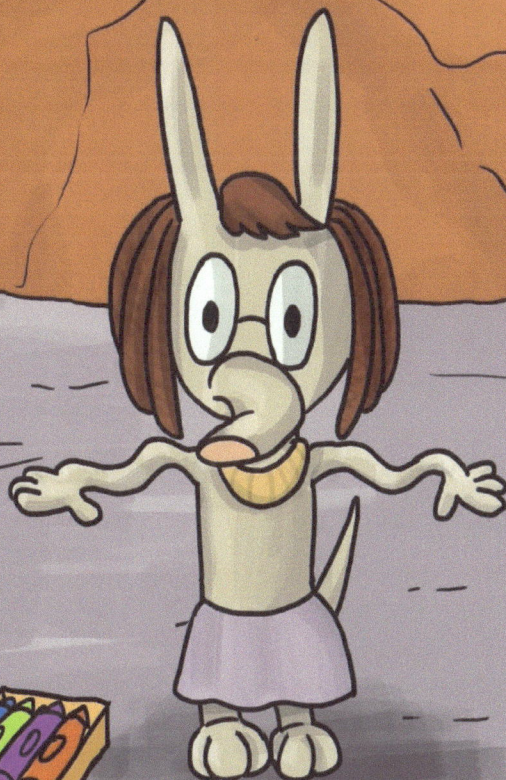

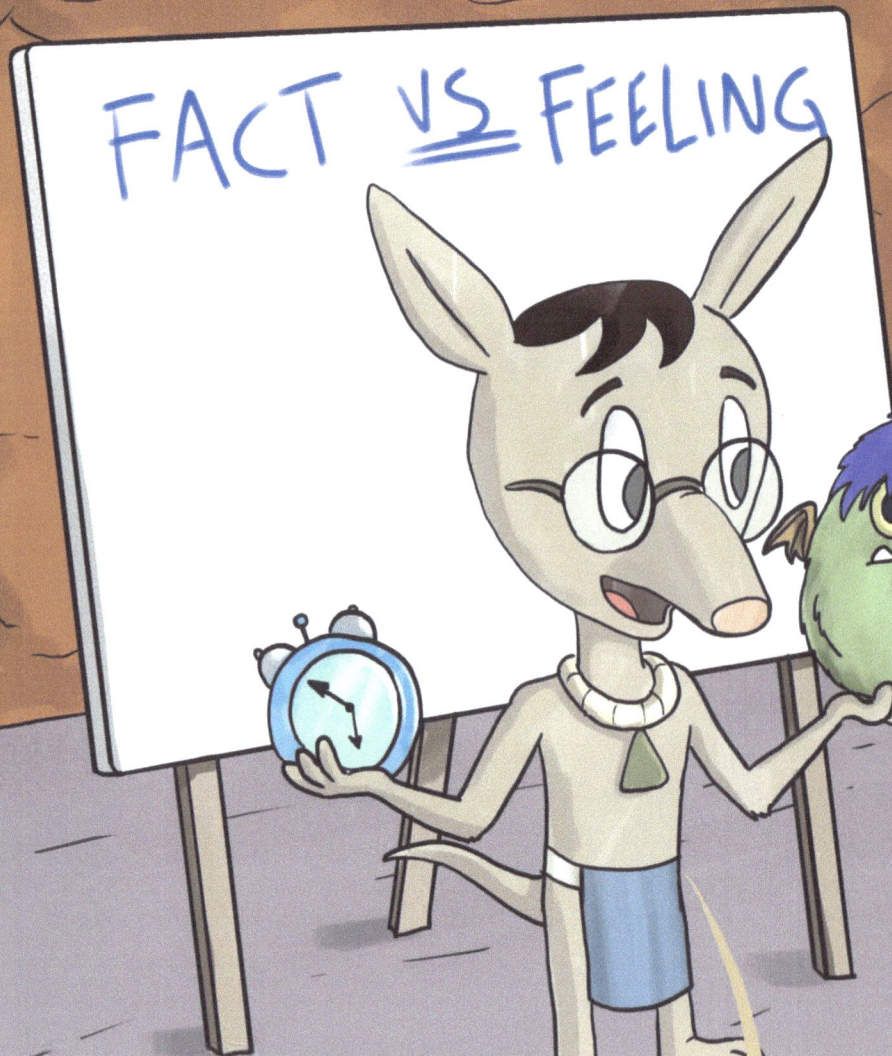

For example, Ayo holds a clock and exclaims:

Remember a clock shows facts: you can't question time because it's known.
On the other hand, a feeling from a monster is just an emotion.
We cannot change a fact, but we can change a feeling, right?

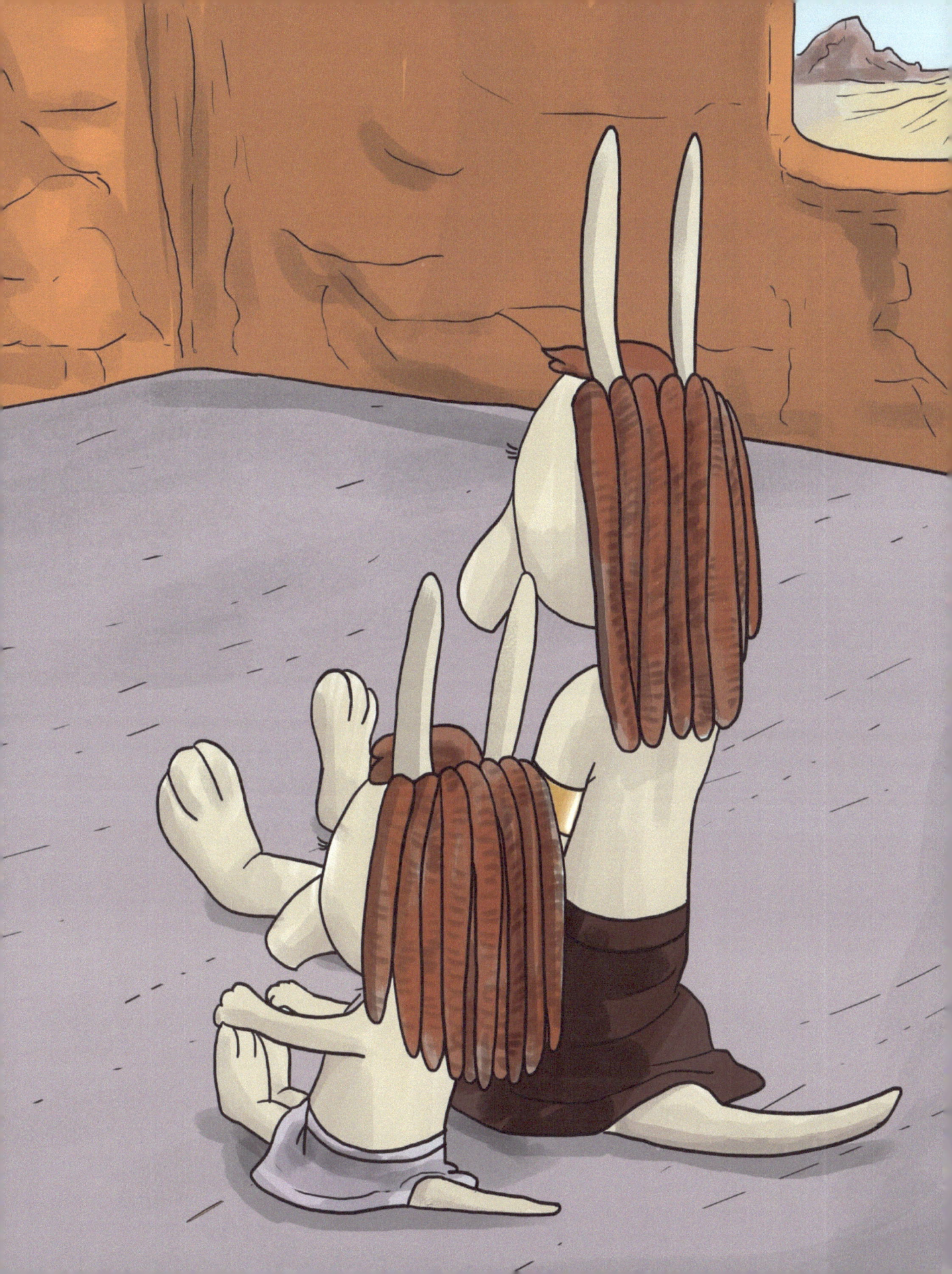

Eager to try this cool trick,
Ace admits,

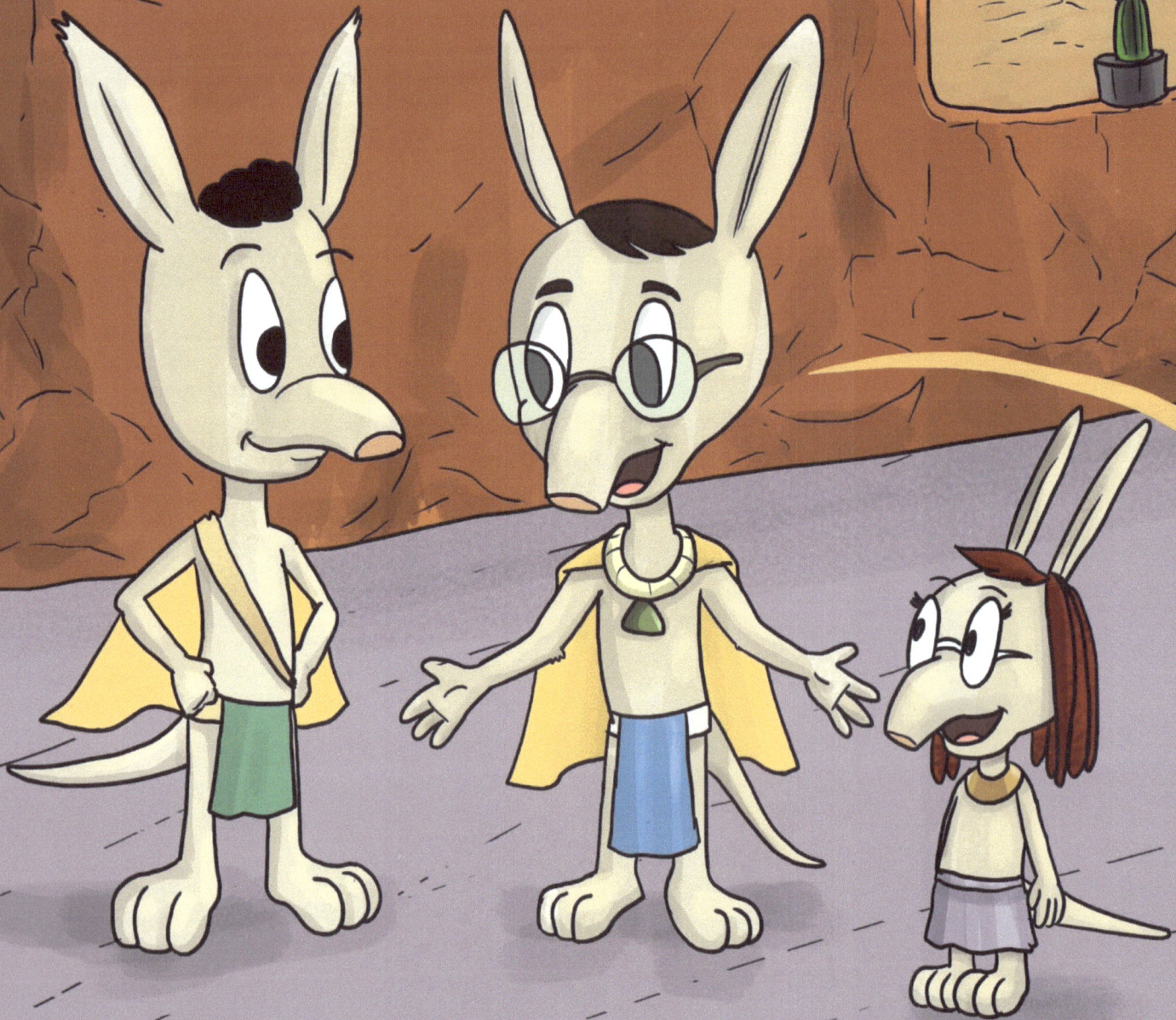

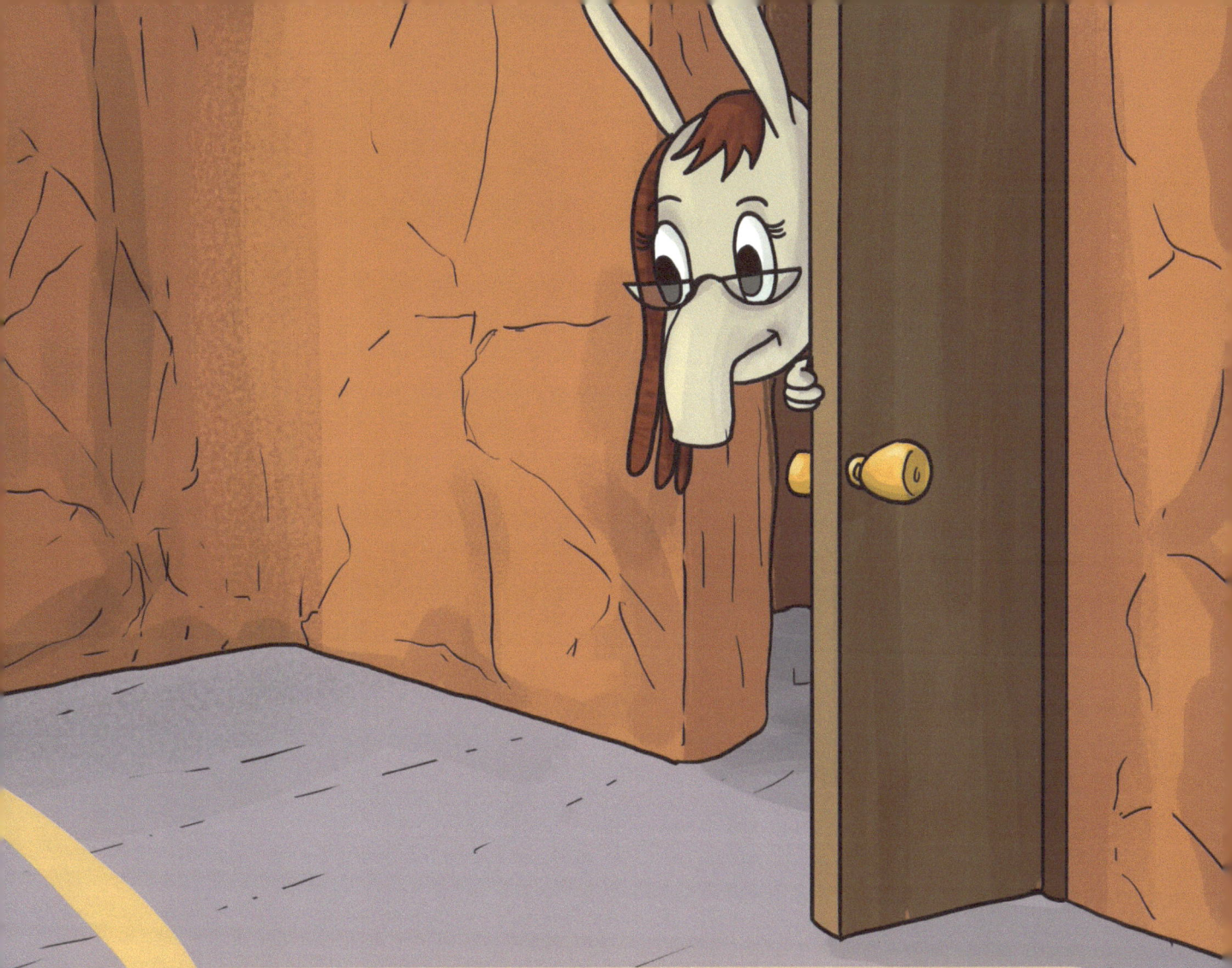

It's a fact that I need to eat to keep my body strong, but it's only my feeling that the termite granola is grainy or scary.

It's also a fact that sand is made of rocks and minerals, yet it's only a fearful feeling that sand will hurt me.

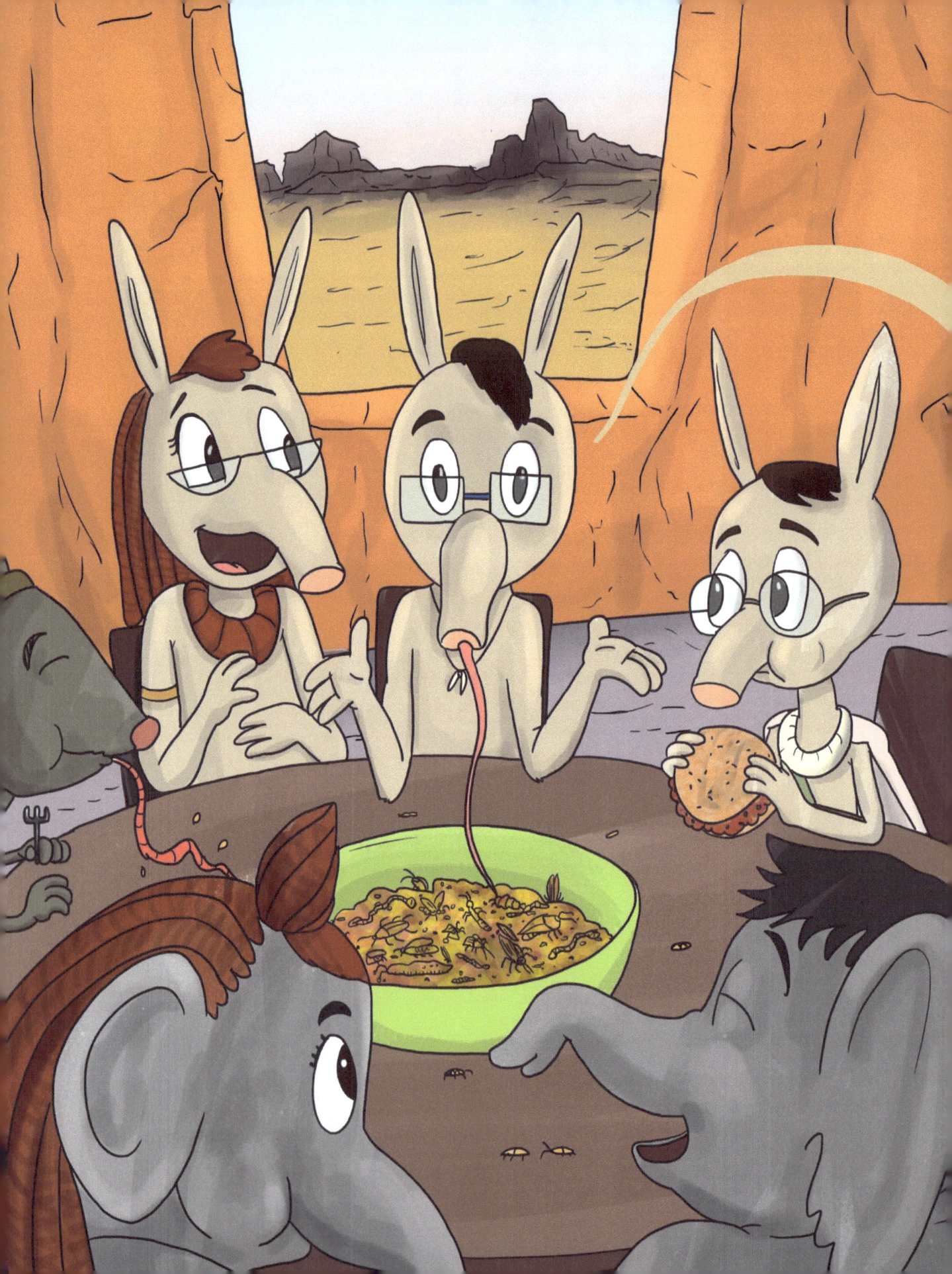

Following more practice and play, Ace is ready for a delightful dinner.

He uses negative thought stopping first, cheerfully chewing his ant burger, and then discussing his worried feelings about sand.

Everyone is proud that he knows it's a feeling versus a fact.

Daddy interrupts with a story:

Son, I once feared worms until I did the feeling versus fact game. It's a FACT that they taste fantastic!

They all giggle and slurp loudly.

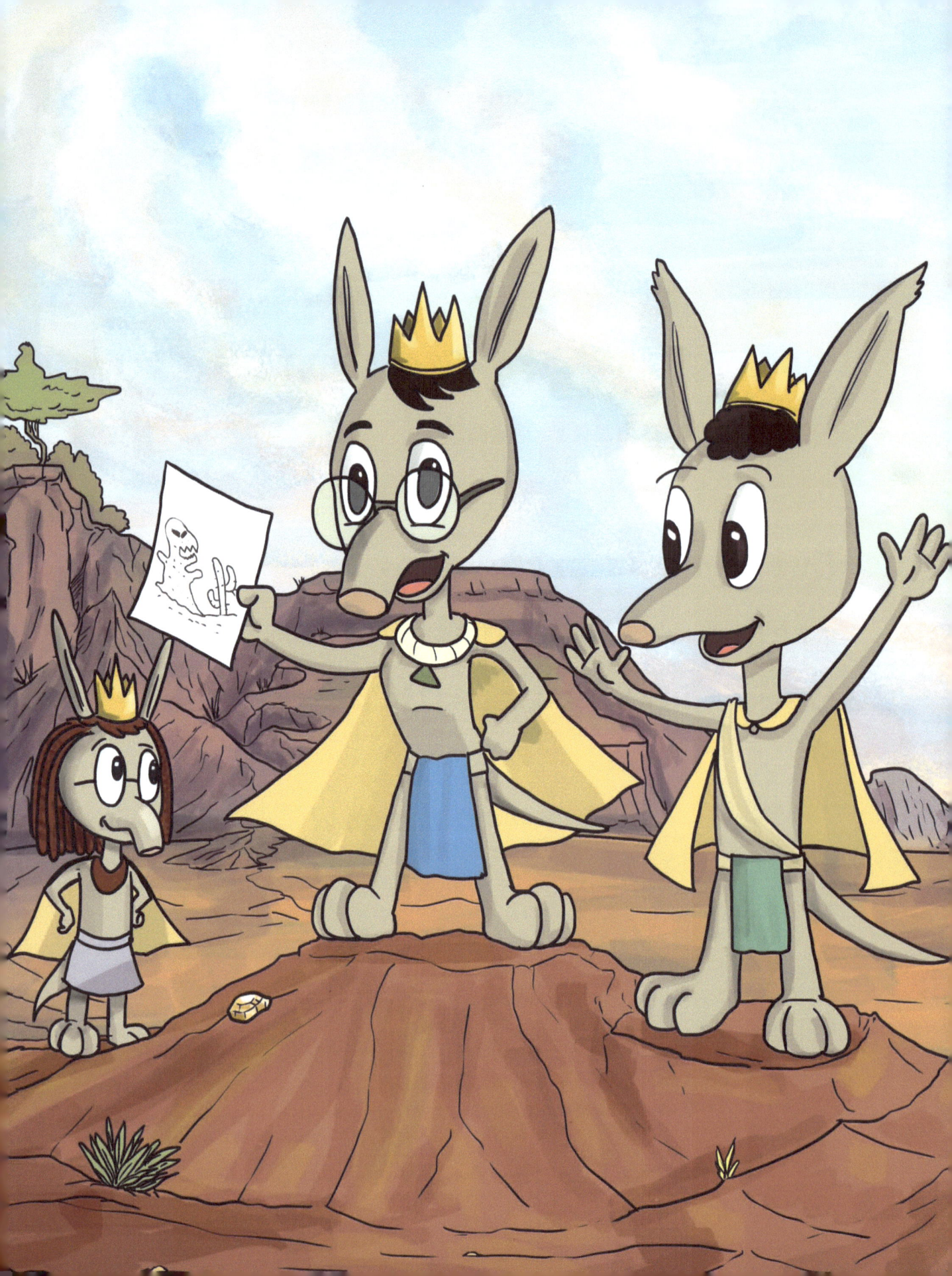

In the end, they watch the sunset over Namibia's dreamy Damaraland.

King Ace eventually freezes his fears of textures as he aces negative thought stopping, calms himself through drawing, gains confidence by talking to his royal "knights," and coping with his challenges using the "facts versus feelings" game.

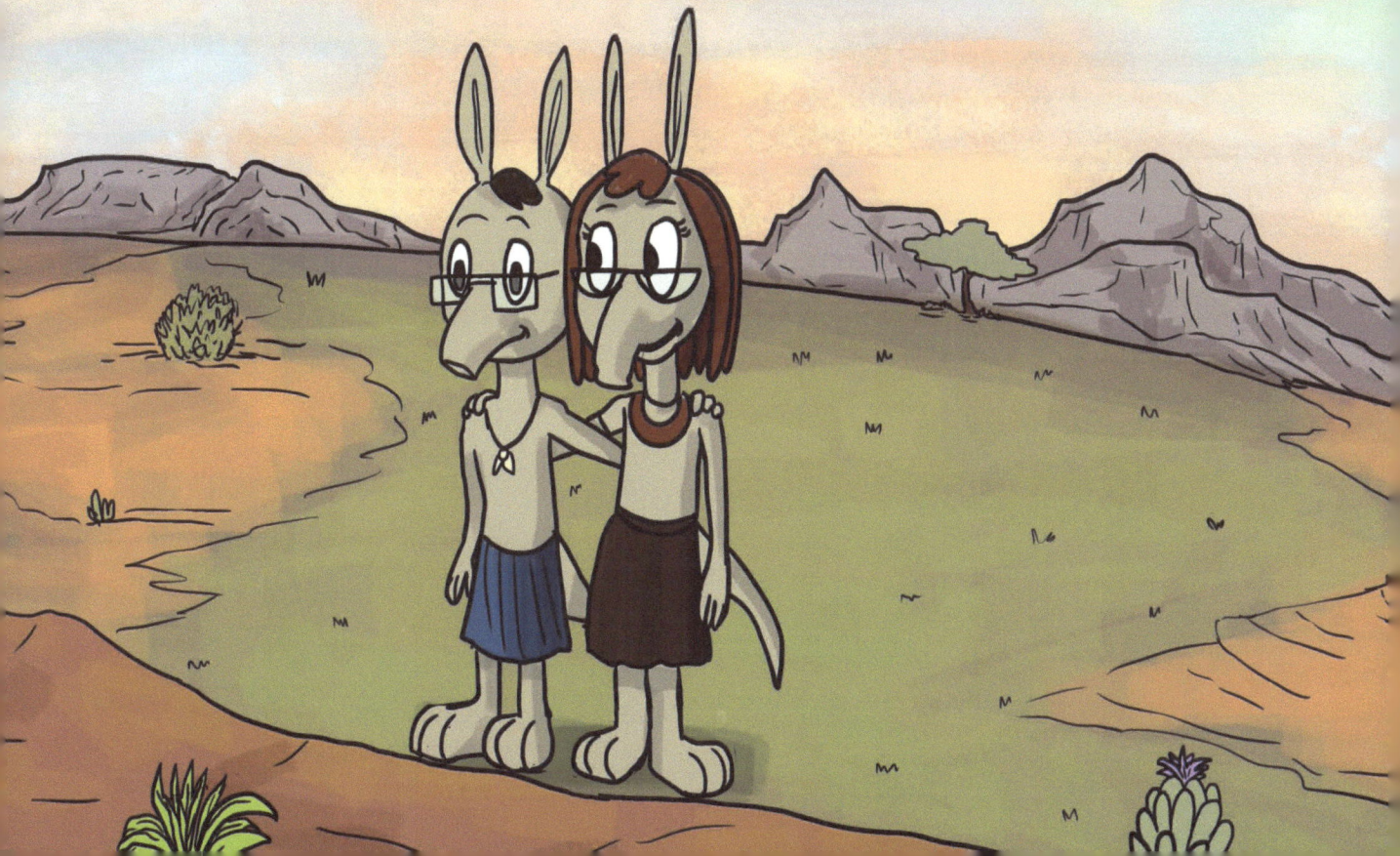

If this King of Courage can make strides over his fears, then try these tips yourself to ace self-control, cope with sensory processing challenges, and gain confidence in your own life as well

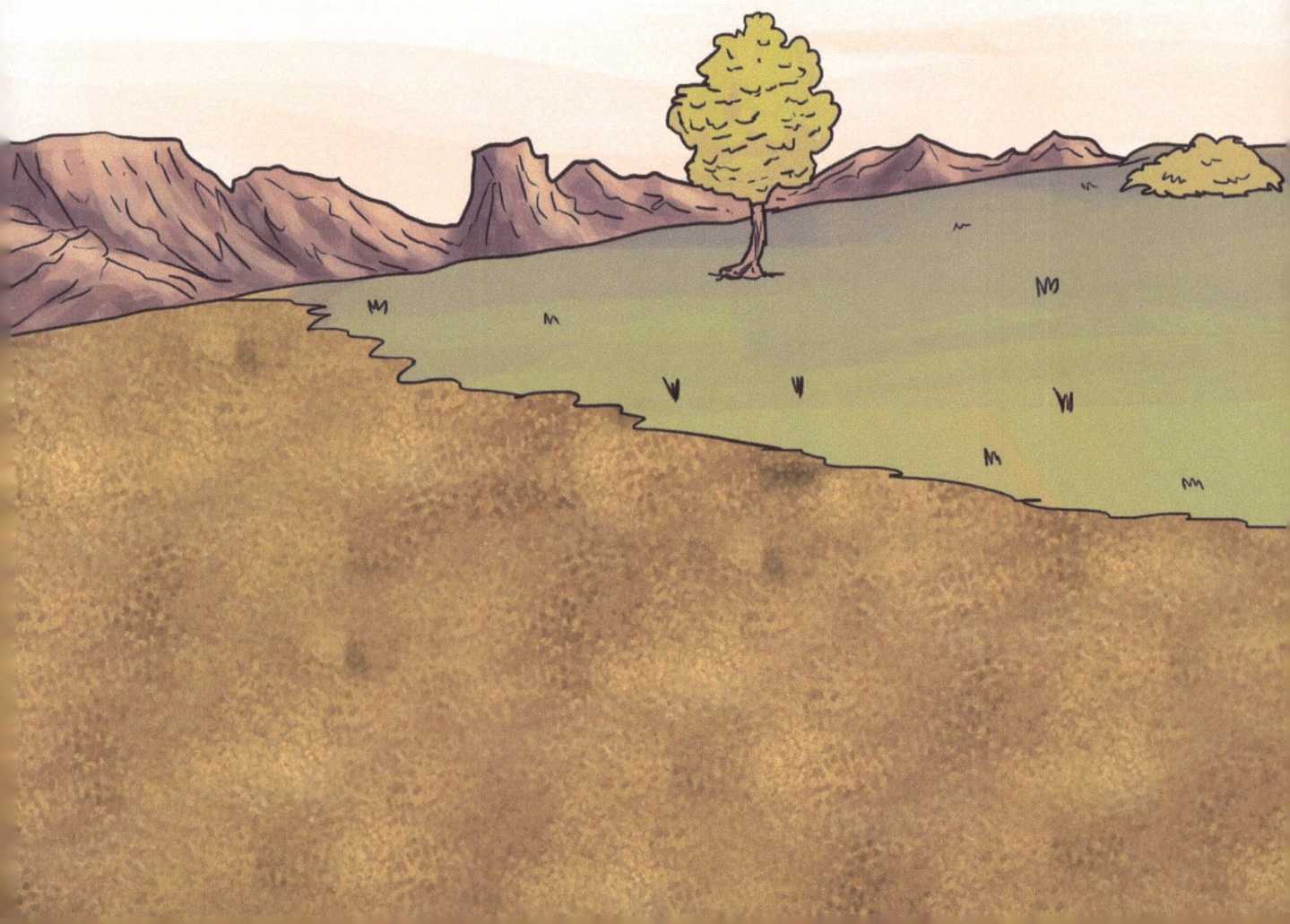

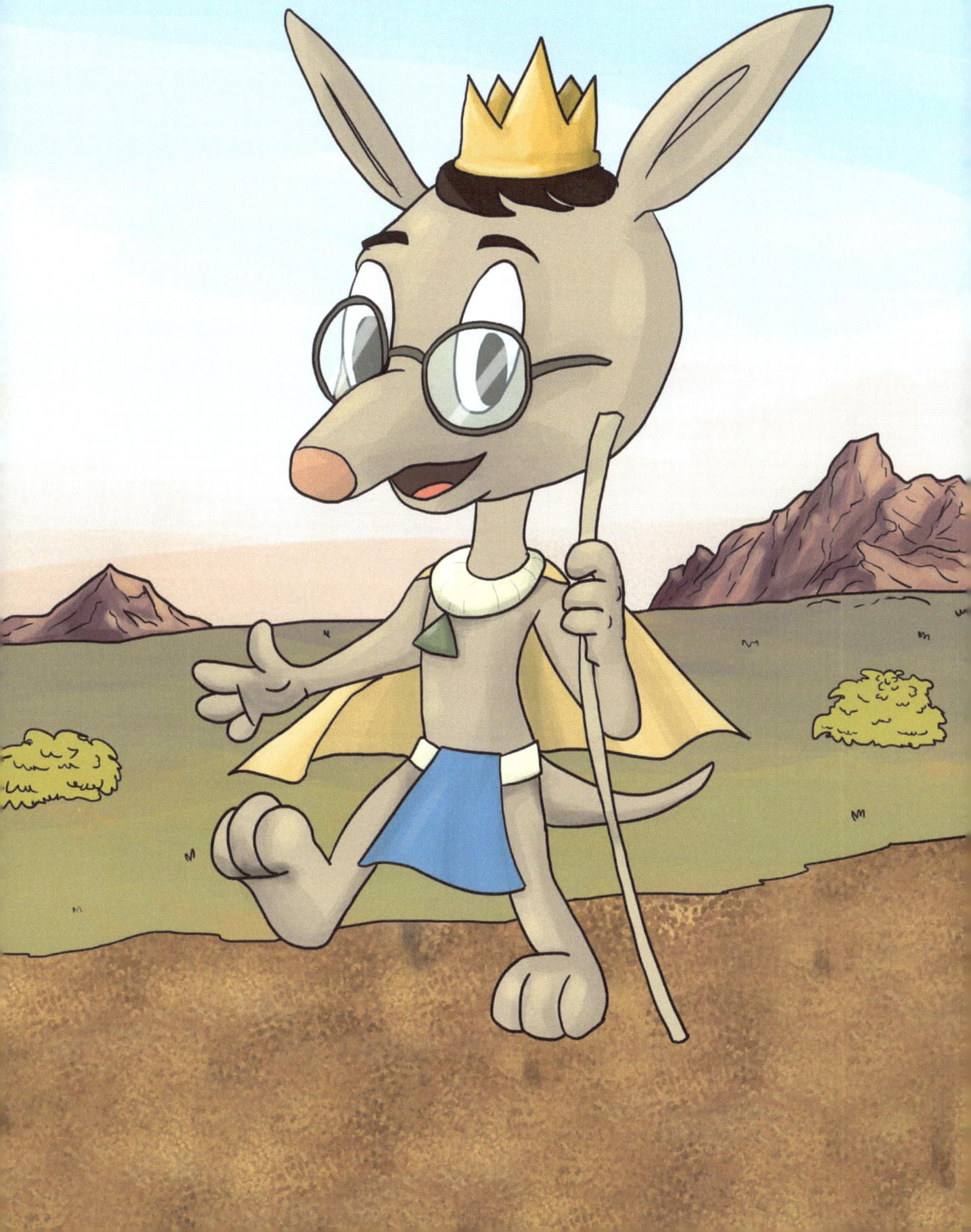

Bonus Post-Reading Activities, Enrichments and Family Fun

1. Virtual African Trip: Name the setting from this book. Then go online with the help of a grownup and locate 4-6 fun facts about this country, culture, its animals, natural resources, languages, customs, religions, history, etc. Fly high with geography!

2. Fact vs. Feeling Game: Think of 2-4 fears that you often have. Practice freezing them like Ace and Ayo did. Did this game help you? How? Teach it to another person today and gain self-control!

3. Fear Jar: Draw or make a fear jar and draw 4-6 things that you fear. Next, place them inside. By naming your fears and locking them inside, try and take comfort that you've taken a big first step to conquer your fears, just like Ace did! This activity pairs with how drawing helps Ace, Ava, and Mom to cope with fears!

4. Aardvark Park: Imagine that you're hired as a park ranger to protect aardvarks. Scan the book again and list 4-6 important facts that you've learned about them from Ace's tale. Soar with science!

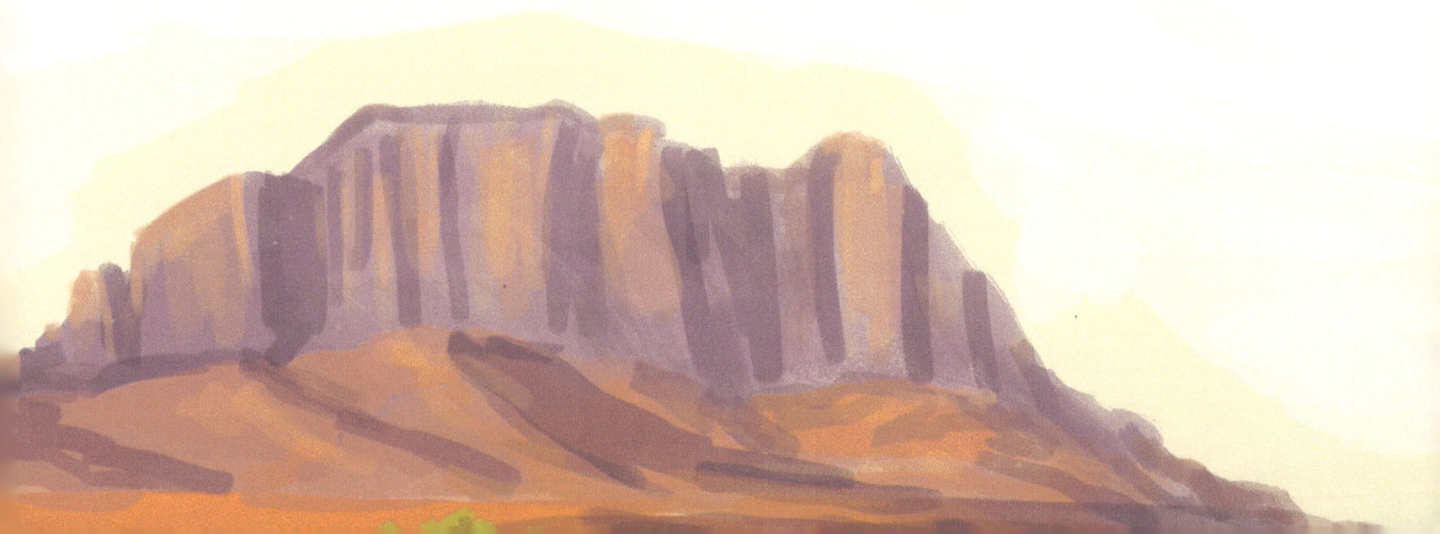

5. Sensory Serenade: What does it mean to have sensory issues or challenges in life?
Have you ever felt like Ace? How did you manage your fears, thoughts, and behaviors?
Grow with confidence over any sensory challenges that make you struggle or stressed.

6. Life Troop: Like Ace's friends and family members who support him, list 4-6 teachers, neighbors, professionals, family members, friends, and coaches who are part of your life troop. Who supports you socially and emotionally?

7. Word Wings: Jot down 4-6 new vocabulary words learned from the book. Define them in your own words before comparing your inferences to a dictionary definition with a family member. Practice saying and spelling them as well for ELA wings.

8. Character MVP: Which character is your favorite? Why? Rock your reading today!

9. Art from the Heart: Which illustration was your favorite? Why?

10. Rhyme Game: Locate 4-6 pairs of rhyming words from the book. Then play a game where you and your friends or family add to these end rhymes and practice this fun ELA skill.

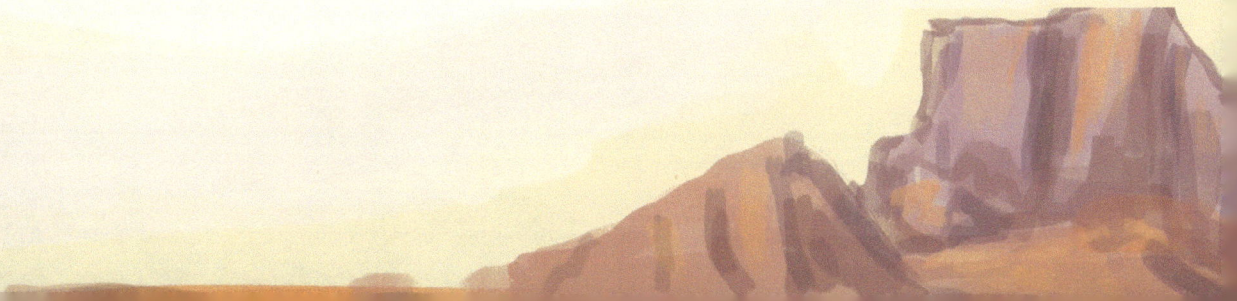

About The Author

After obtaining her BS in Secondary English Education and MA in English from Slippery Rock University of PA, Stacy embarked on a successful teaching career that spanned public, government, and charter schools in Pittsburgh, PA, Oklahoma City, Norman, OK, and Okinawa, Japan.

She proudly earned a 2004 Fulbright-Hays Seminar Scholarship to Thailand and Vietnam from the United States Department of Education, Teacher of the Year in two schools, as well as other teaching accolades.

However, her greatest achievements involved collaborating with other inspiring teachers and staff, meeting amazing families, and also interacting with memorable and diverse students who taught her so much about life and humanity!

In addition to multicultural and social activism, Stacy savors sweet moments with her awesome husband, two fierce and fabulous daughters, and three frisky fur babies. She presently works as a virtual freelancer, private English and ESL tutor, and online editor/proofreader. When she's not book buzzing, Stacy enjoys films, travel, books, coffee, art, and all things mindful!

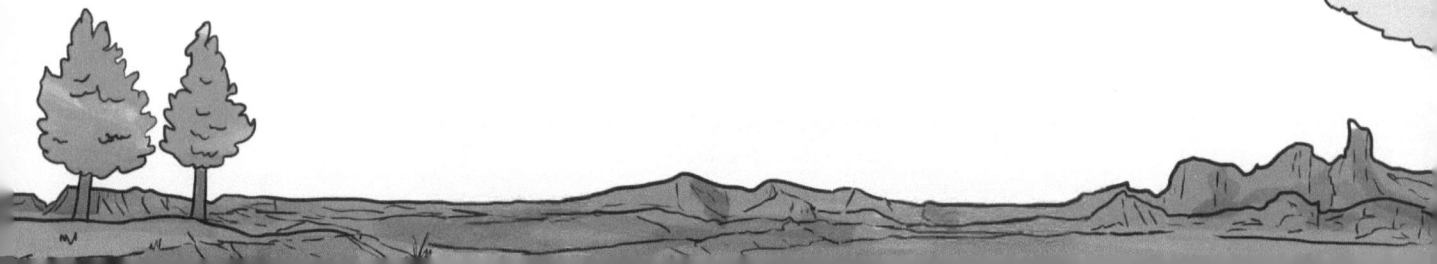

About the Illustrator

Danko Herrera studied Industrial Design in Mexico and Denmark and after spending a sabbatical year backpacking, he started his own short tales collection with the help of the art collective Sombrerero, which he founded with his travel friends.

Danko continues on the freelance illustration bussiness up to this day, helping authors create their universe with pixels and brushes. Danko has worked with a variety of authors and companies such as Rockademix, Indie Publishing Group, Process Cat, Jeff Rivera and Arnie Lightning.

Besides illustration, he loves traveling, studies the ancient egyptian language, plays the clarinet and didgeridoo and can do the throat singing.

You can visit Danko's website and follow on Instagram

http://danko.mx

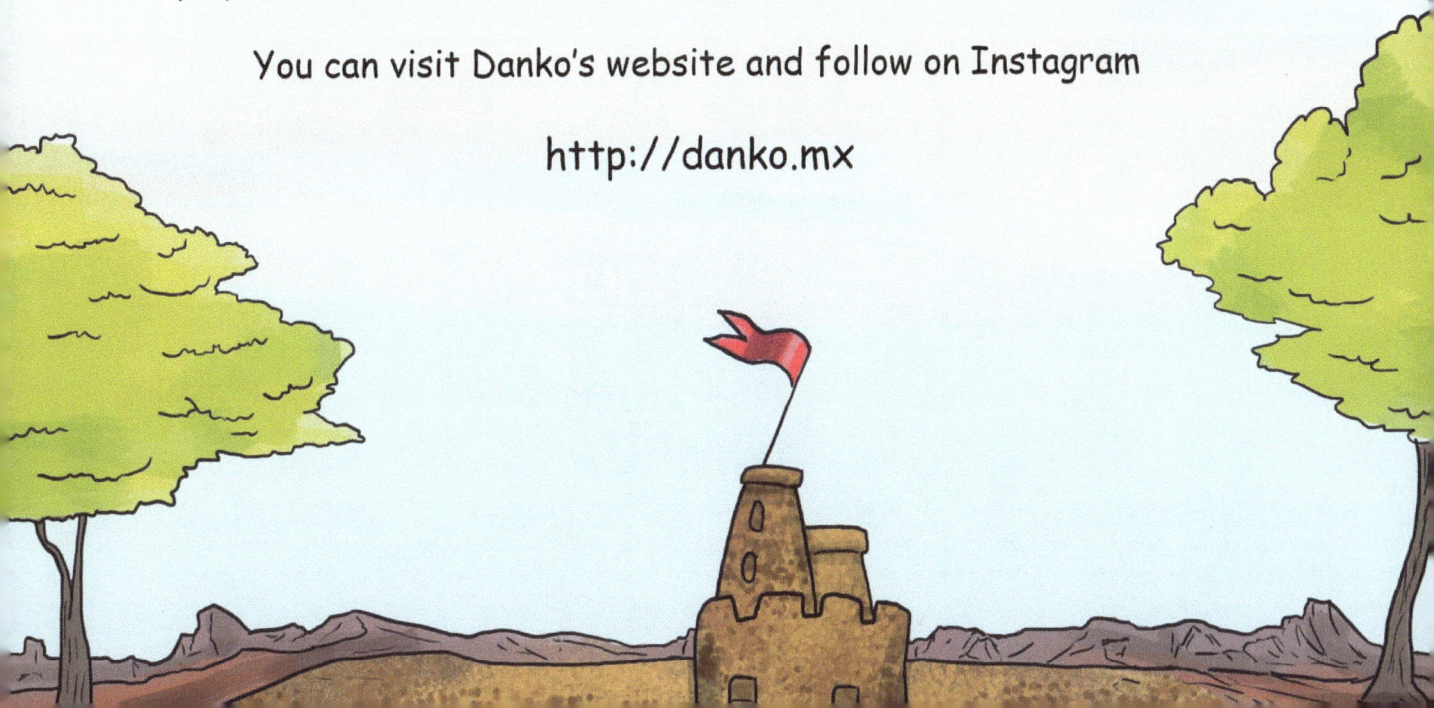

Thank you for buying this book.

As a working mom and military spouse, your reviews mean so much to me because I aim to unite global readers through art and literacy.

Kindly post a short review on this book's Amazon page.
I truly appreciate your time to book buzz with me!
If you like this book, then please check out my others at

https://www.amazon.com/Stacy-Shaneyfelt/e/B08TVX7C5X/

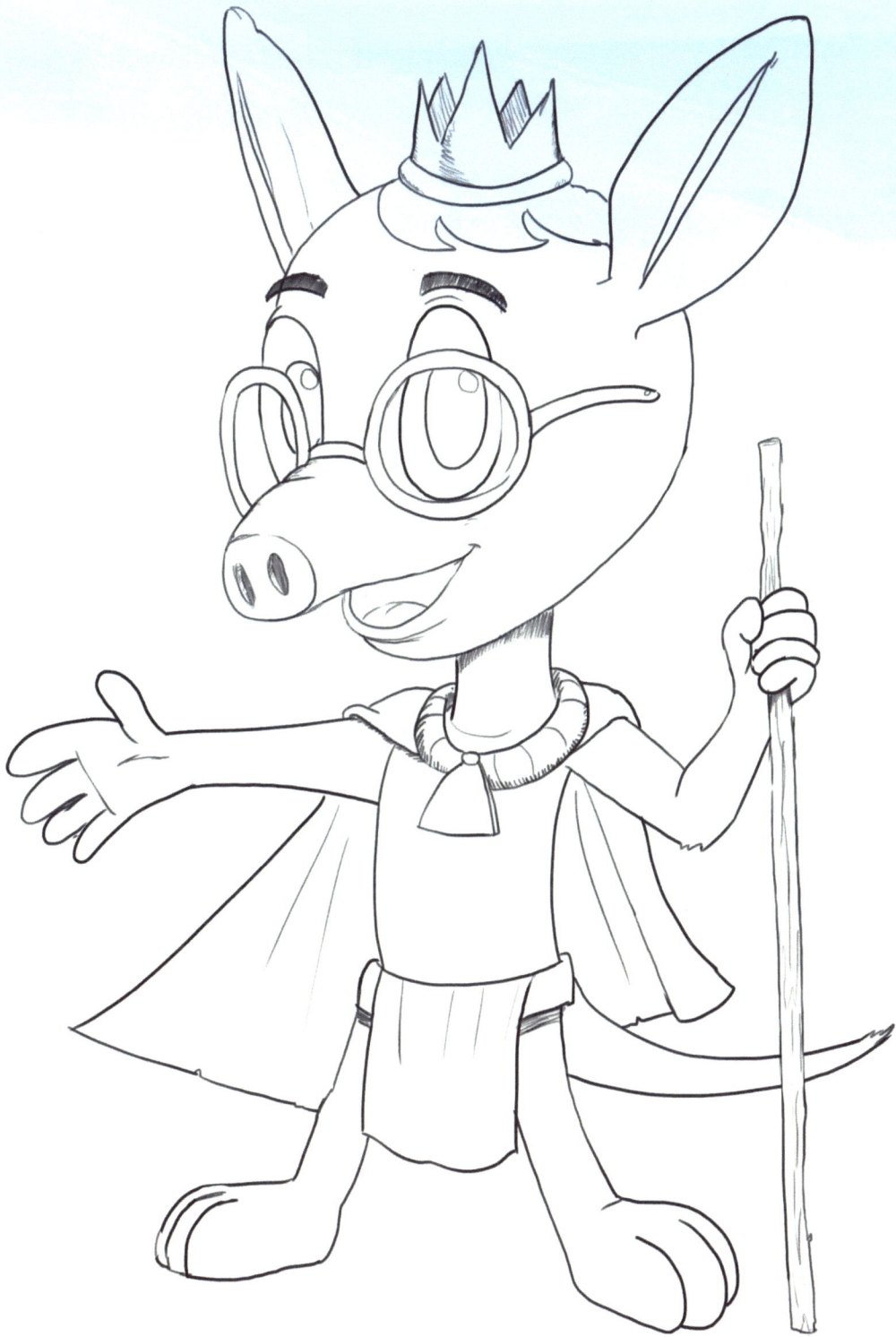

www.ingramcontent.com/pod-product-compliance
Lightning Source LLC
Chambersburg PA
CBHW060853270326
41934CB00002B/123